More naked than other people

Marijn van der Jagt

In the TV series Sex and the City, when Samantha was found to have breast cancer, she and her three girlfriends didn't see it as a reason to be gloomy. They just moved their gatherings from the club to the clinic where Samantha lay on the drip, receiving chemotherapy. The women sat on their chaise longue chatting away as if they were sitting in a beauty parlour. They gossiped, chatted about sex and sipped drinks. Rosy cheeks, trendy clothes, red lipstick and perfectly coiffeured hair: the façade of eternal beauty was kept up even in the chemotherapy clinic. The panic only came later, when in the same installment of the series Samantha held a large tuft of her beautiful blond hair in her hand. Well, actually, first it was Samantha's stripling of a lover who looked with surprise at her hair in his hand. The kinky scene in which that happened typified the trail-blazing frivolity with which Sex and the City handled carnal desire. The loss of hair took place during an undisguised bout of lovemaking, and you saw the young man think for just a moment that he had pulled the hair from Samantha's head in pure passion. But the terror in her eyes, and the rapid gesture with which she grabs her hair back – 'Just give that here!' – makes it clear that this loss of hair was coupled with a shameful loss of face. The snogging was over, the lover is shown the door. In the privacy of her bathroom Samantha takes the scissors to shear off her blond locks.

It was an uncompromising act for a woman who (at least in the TV series) needed the attractive appearance of hair. Yet every TV viewer understood why Samantha did it. Rather a self-chosen bald 'cut' than the risk of losing hair in public. However hip the shaving off of hair from various places on the body may be at the moment, that same hair falling out remains a taboo. Monique Benthin, the initiator of the photography project of which this book is a part, has hardly any photographs of herself from the periods that she was bald. Like all other bearers of the condition alopecia areata, her baldness – whether localised or complete, periodic or protracted – is not self-chosen. The issue is not the being bald, but the becoming bald; and people today have no positive associations with the latter.

It is the natural process of change that we have problems with. The growth of hair where it is unwanted can fill us with repulsion, and many a horror film seizes upon that anxiety by showing the growth process speeded up. Body hair symbolises the difference between humans and animals, between men and women, between children and adults, and the down with which babies – particularly premature babies – come into the world is a hold-over from a primaeval age with which we no longer wish to be associated. Every day, in television adverts, magazines and advertising posters, we are adjured to keep its growth in various places under control. Men flaunt their smooth chests, women stroke their stubble-free legs, minimalist slipsshow that the 'bikini line' encompasses more than just the inside of the thighs, and in Viva's (Dutch women's magazine) nude bodies feature 'Any body', all crotches under the age of forty are subject to a drastic deforestation. These are all proofs of decisiveness. Here civilised man triumphs over brute nature.

When it comes to head hair, the adjurations of the cosmetic industry are reversed. The hair on our heads is the flowerbed of the garden that is our body. On other parts of our body, the weeds must be constantly checked; on the head, every means must be used to promote the growth and flourishing of hair. For the hair on our heads there is only one rule, which transcends all eras and fashions. It must be full, and cover all; for women, it should preferably be long. In the Bible, the Pentateuch already contains a precise guide that prescribes how the growth of hair must be encouraged, and its dropping out discouraged. The hair of your head must not decrease. It must grow and multiply. If necessary, this must happen artificially, with painfully woven-in 'dreads' or through humiliating hair implants. The positive associations of a full head of hair are more than just symbolic. The hair on our heads is a gauge of our health. The growth of our hair reflects the vitality of our body. 'Hair renews itself much more spectacularly than skin, nails or teeth,' writes Inge Stephan in the collection Körperteile (Rowolt, 2001). 'Even continuous cutting or shaving will not disrupt its continuous, life-long growth.' Hormonal changes or the use of medicines, or our psychological well-being: these however can have an immediate effect on the condition of our hair. Those who carry alopecia areata know stress can cause hair to fall out. This knowledge leaves them extra 'naked' at moments when the illness strikes. With the bald spots on their heads they not only run counter to every idea of what is fashionable, but also indirectly expose a part of their internal state.

In films the loss of large tufts of hair is a favourite means of depicting an inward crisis. With the tuft of her hair, Samantha's stripling of a lover in Sex and the City had the most vulnerable side of his indomitable sex partner in his hands. That he catches her a bit later in the bathroom at work with the shears was the litmus test of his character and of their relation. He could have taken to his heels in shock, but instead of doing that he takes the electric shaver and shows his involvement in her drama through a sacrifice of his own. Before her astonished eyes the young god also shaves off his own blond locks. At the end of the instalment the viewers see the attractive pair stepping out of their limousine at one media event or another. He is flaunting his newly shaven head. She has her bald head hidden under a curly lavender wig.

Going bald is not the same for men and women. For most men, the loss of hair on their head will be unavoidable. Fashion at the moment dictates camouflaging that process as much as possible – many hair experts on television have already pronounced a ban on simply covering a balding skull by combing the hair across it. Still, a man who does not abide by this is not a curiosity to be stared at. But a bald woman is. For her, shaving her head completely is not an option either. After all, there are very few examples of women who present a bald head as an ideal of beauty. No matter how beautiful bald women might be when they appear in the media, they are sinister extraterrestrials, butch mavericks or militant street fighters. The sudden baldness of singer Sinéad O'Connor was in its time a progressive change of image, such as Madonna had already undergone dozens of times. Yet videoclip viewers saw her new style as an expression of rage and despair. Today's woman has a free choice of many images and roles - but her choosing to shave her hair off is experienced as a protest. A man's hair symbolises his strength and his potency. The Biblical hero Samson immediately lost his preternatural strength when his hair was cut off. Even today, in contemporary films, mythic heroes often have long hair. A woman's hair stands for her sexuality. She can indeed perform deeds of strength with it, as Rapunzel does in the fairy tale, when she has her rescuers climb up her long tresses. But ultimately Rapunzel's hair is more a highway than a weapon: anyone who follows this princess's hair will possess her in the most intimate way. The hair on a woman's head, and also the hair under her arms, refers to the hair that covers her most secret spot. That women with alopecia areata can lose their hair in all these charged places makes them vulnerable in still another way: they fall outside the physical code of revealing and covering, referring to and keeping secret. Under their clothing they are more naked than other people.

Right to the present day, for women long hair is the fulfilment of desire. Little girls dream of having long hair. The cosmetics industry kisses this little girl's dream awake daily among adult women, with advertisements in which their beautiful compatriots let their hair fly around them in slow motion. It is a visual mantra that hypnotises men and seduces women to purchase still more hair care products. That women in many cultures are required to cover their hair confirms the sexual power that is attributed to the hair on the head. Among orthodox Jewish women, the natural hair is even shaved off to make way for a more controllable head covering: the wig.

Therefore it is not strange that Samantha's young lover in Sex and the City responds to her cutting off her hair with an act of his own. The fact is that the shaving of Samantha's blond locks also had significance in the balance of power in their relationship. She deprives herself of one of the most attractive parts of her body – but she also deprives him of it too. The scene in the bathroom, with the tufts of shaved-off hair in the sink, put one in mind of a painting by Frida Kahlo, her self-portrait from 1940 entitled Autorretrato con pelo cortado. Kahlo shows herself shortly after she cut off her beautiful long hair, which she always artfully put up on her head and decorated with bows and flowers. The hair she has cut off writhes around on the floor next to the chair in which she sits, scissors in hand. It seems to have taken possession of the room, weeds which have been torn up out a flowerbed. Even when cut off, the hair testifies to a vitality; if it were to be preserved, it might easily outlive Kahlo herself. Kahlo could make a wig of it, a 'hairpiece' such as was made in the 19th century, or perhaps an item of clothing, like the hair dresses and blouses that the Korean artist Elaine Kim makes for bald models. It is a marvellous way of returning their hair to hairless people.

The Mexican painter has depicted herself in a man's suit, a reference to the distinction between men and women in which hair is such a decisive factor. Above her portrait Kahlo has written two lines from a Mexican folk song: 'Look, when I loved you it was because of your hair. / Now that you are shaven bald, I no longer love you.' With this painting Kahlo was dealing with her own feelings about her husband's adultery. But it was also a message to the adulterous man, from whose lustful gaze she was withdrawing one of her feminine characteristics. With this painting, Kahlo is showing us not only her despair, but also her power - power over her sexual aura, over her own appearance. With her new 'hairdo' Kahlo – like Samantha in Sex and the City - is creating a new image of herself. That is what people generally use their hair for; our hair style is one of the means by which we make a statement about our individuality. The hair on their heads is important for the image that people have of themselves, and the image that others have of them. It contributes to the 'staging of the I', as Inge Stephan writes in Körperteile. All over the world, the shaving off of hair is used to deprive people – monks, military conscripts, war prisoners – of their individuality. That is what makes the 'ordinary' head shaving because of a hair disease or hair loss so frustrating. It deprives the bald-shaven person of the possibility of expressing his or her identity. But anyone looking at Frida Kahlo in her painting, after she has cut her hair short, sees no identityless being. Quite the contrary: Kahlo is revealing just how much personality and individual beauty has been hidden under her long hair. By means of this image Kahlo is seizing a new ground: she is changing herself from a spurned object of desire into a decisive subject.
This turn-around also lies at the heart of the photographs which were made for the project Undercover/Onthecover. Men and women with alopecia areata, who in everyday life are reduced to objects by the surreptitious gaze of the curious, here turn the tables on the others. They show themselves to a photographer, who aestheticises their unusual appearance. They reveal how different they are - and how little hair you actually need for the expression of strength, beauty and personality.

For people with h air, a bit of hai r, or none at al l

Monique Benthin

Why is it that hair and identity are so closely linked with each other? Why do people find that hair contributes to self-confidence, strength and a positive self-image? Hair has always played an important role in the appearance of men and women. It can make you stand out in a crowd, whether you want to or not. Losing a lot of hair is an emotional event.
Undercover/Onthecover: this play on words came to me while I was still only half-awake early one morning in the winter of 2003. In retrospect the words are instinctive, and with respect to their content, were the impetus for organising this photography project, which also finally bears the title Undercover/Onthecover.

I realised how liberating it would be if alopecia areata would become familiar in a way that the people who have to live with it could show themselves as beautiful, healthy and strong men and women. Right down to this present day, undesired baldness is something accompanied by a strong sense of shame, and can be said to be uncommon among women and children. For me, the title symbolises the ambivalent feelings people have to deal with when alopecia areata suddenly appears in their life, briefly or permanently. This still unfamiliar disease of the hair has played a major role in my life and in the lives of many others. People around me didn't find me ugly when I lost all my hair when I was seventeen; indeed they found my hairless head strikingly beautiful. It's just that I didn't want to be bald in this way; I didn't want to be from another planet or a woman from the future.
My image in the mirror and the people around me told me that there was something wrong with me: I was different. In the sight of others, and also in front of my own mirror, I covered up my head, and thereby too - entirely against my will – a great deal of my personality. Although this phenomenon has been around since time immemorial, it is often associated with something which happens in the distant future, as that is shown to us in many science fiction films. As far as I know, no history of hairless people has ever been written. Also, unlike extremely hirsute people - think of the bearded woman - they have never been an object of interest in the circus, fun fair or raree show. Because people are not familiar with the condition, they quickly conclude that your peculiar appearance is something you have consciously chosen, by cutting, shaving or plucking your hair.
I found that the photographers of my choice were prepared to co-operate in putting together the photo exhibition and its accompanying photo book. Their reactions to my request to help give shape to this project with new photographic images were curious and spontaneous, in a positive way. Important factors in choosing them were the high degree of 'vulnerability' inherent to the topic and a necessary respect for the persons being portrayed.
I hope that the photo exhibition and book will be the occasion for new insights into the influence that hair - or its absence - has on our self-image and on the manner in which others see and make judgements about us.

I wish to thank all those who in their distinctive, caring, inspiring and fascinating ways have assisted in realising this project, so valuable for me and many others, both visually and with texts, and with their advice and support.

Also, I would like to thank the people of the Dutch alopecia areata foundation who have made it possible to find the models for this project. At the University of Tilburg, I would like to thank drs Marco Mulders for initiating scientific research of the loss of hair and related well being amongst women.

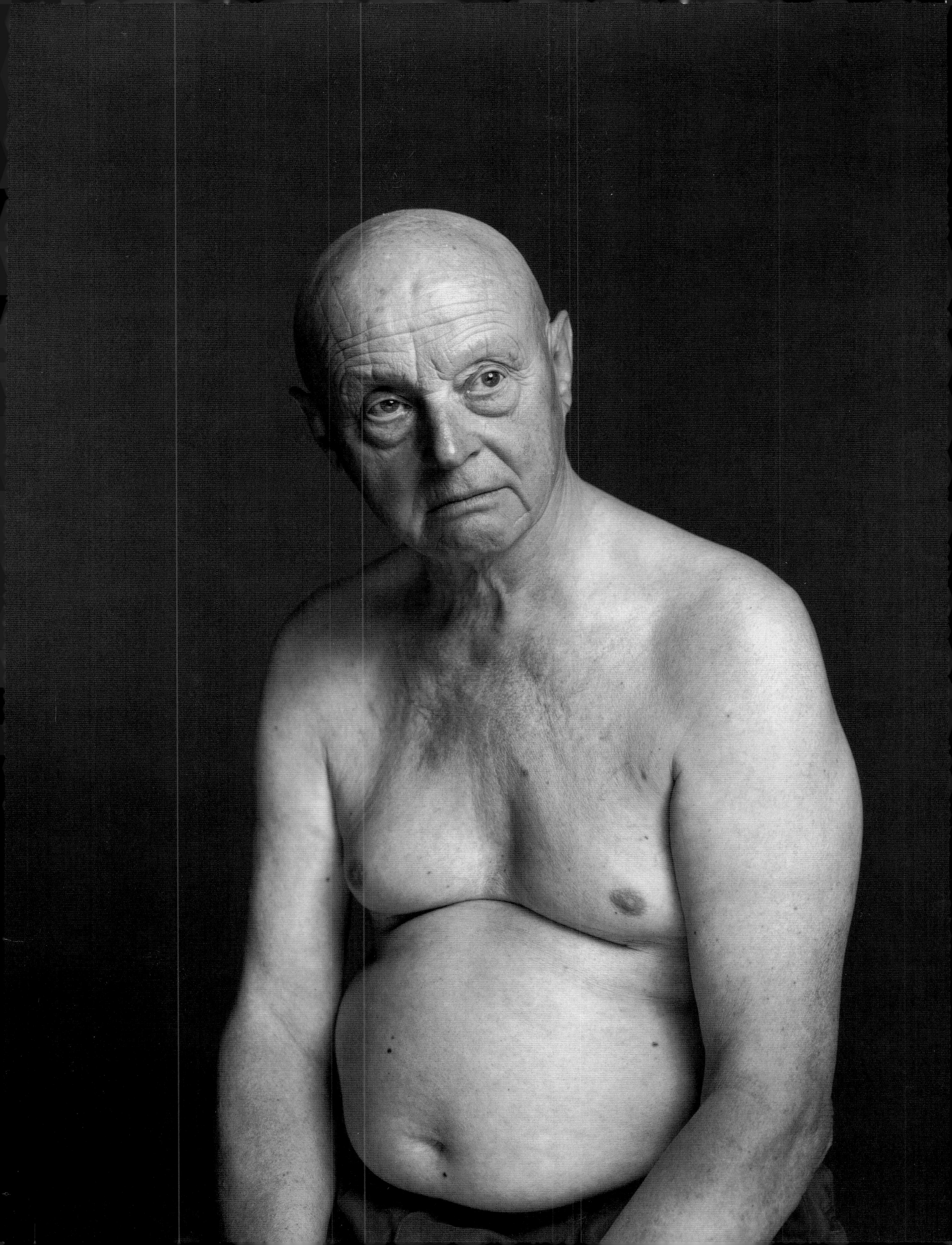

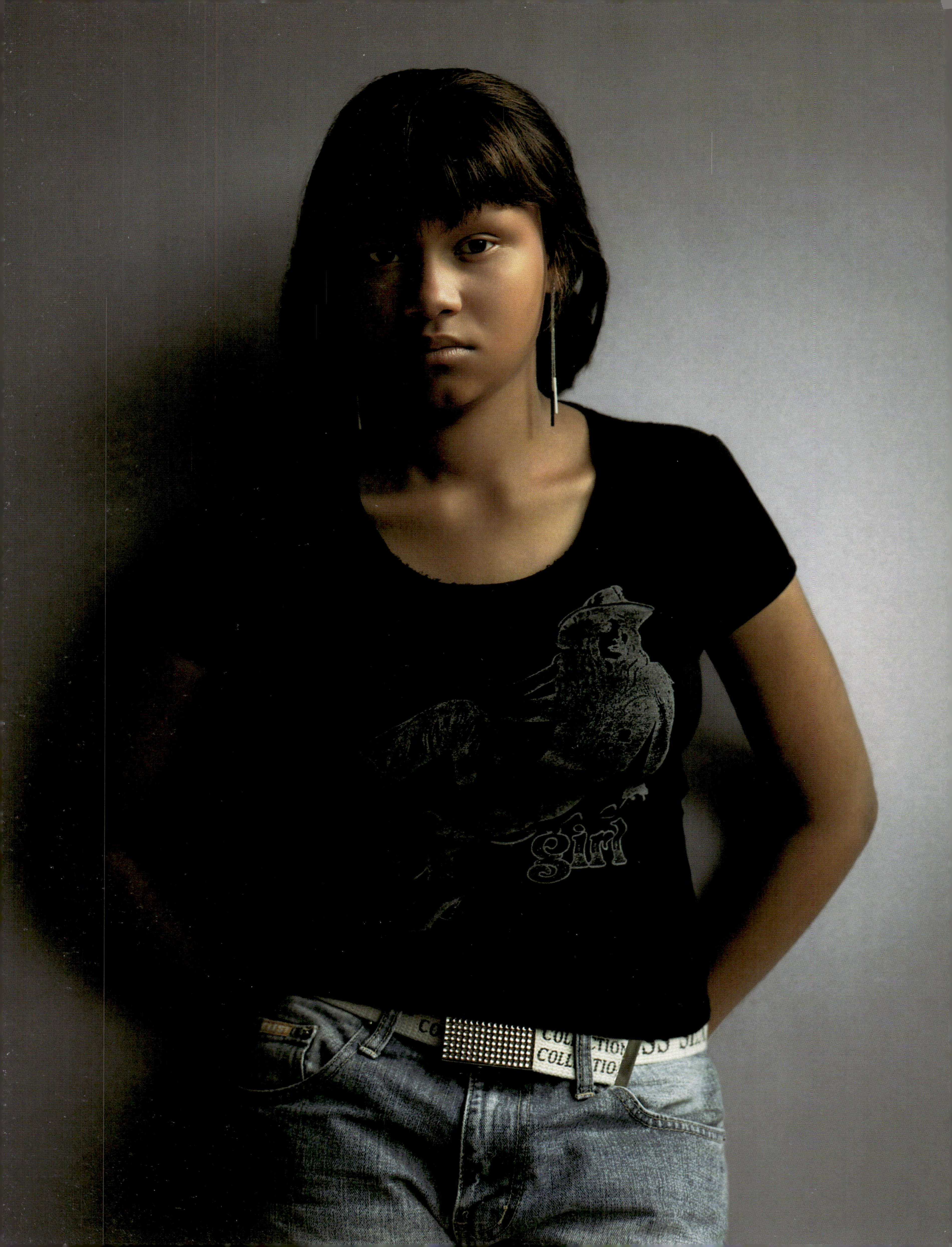
girl

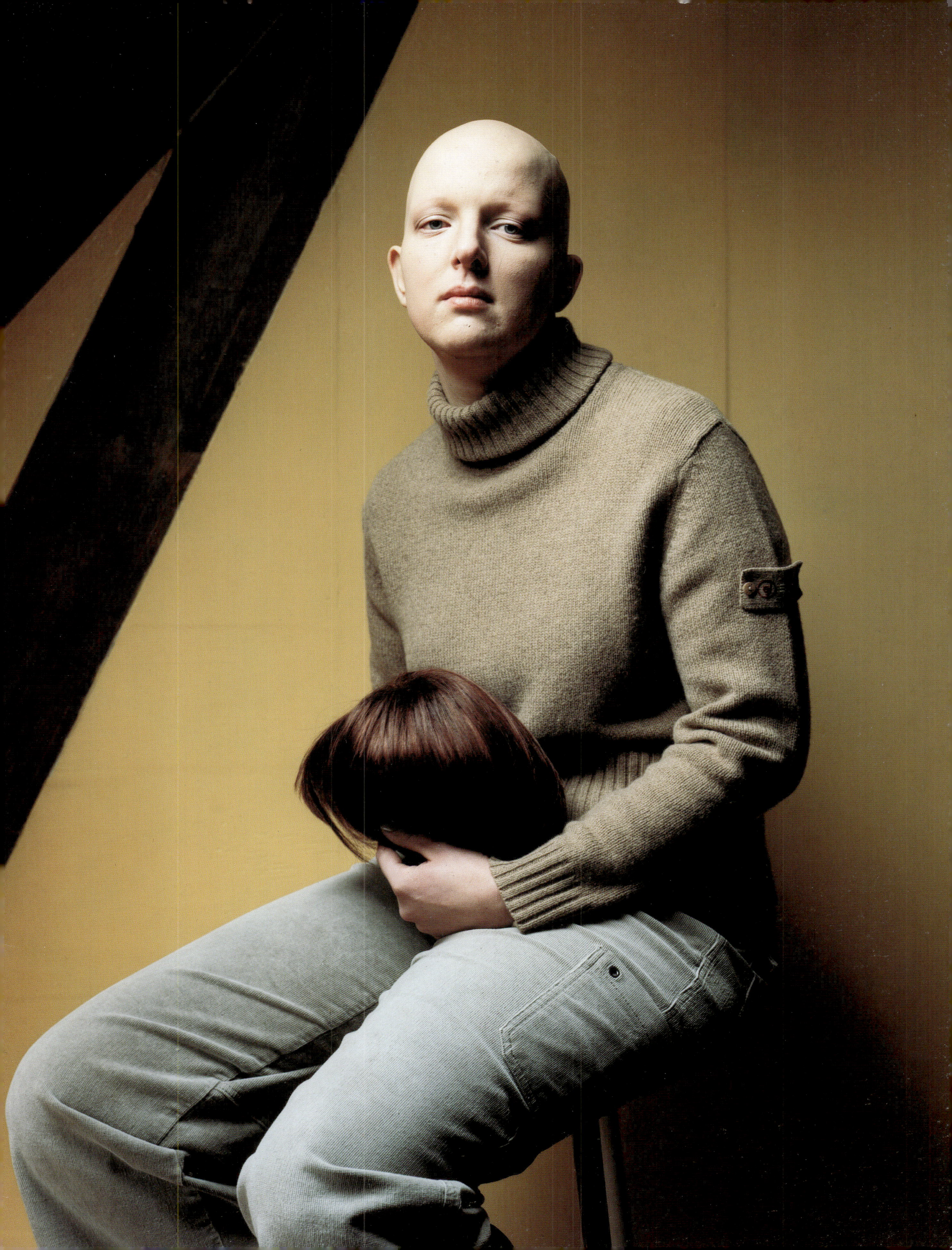

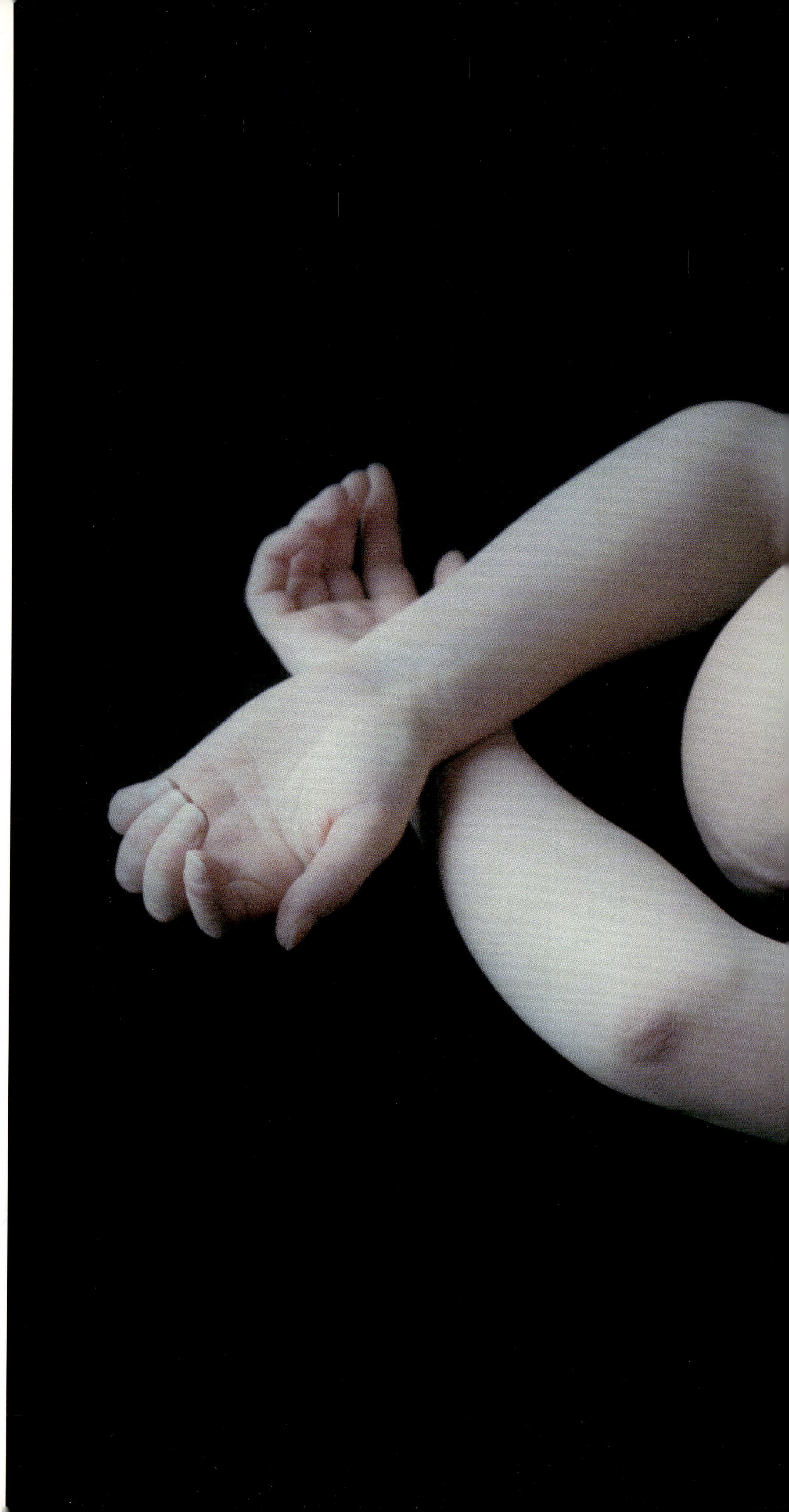

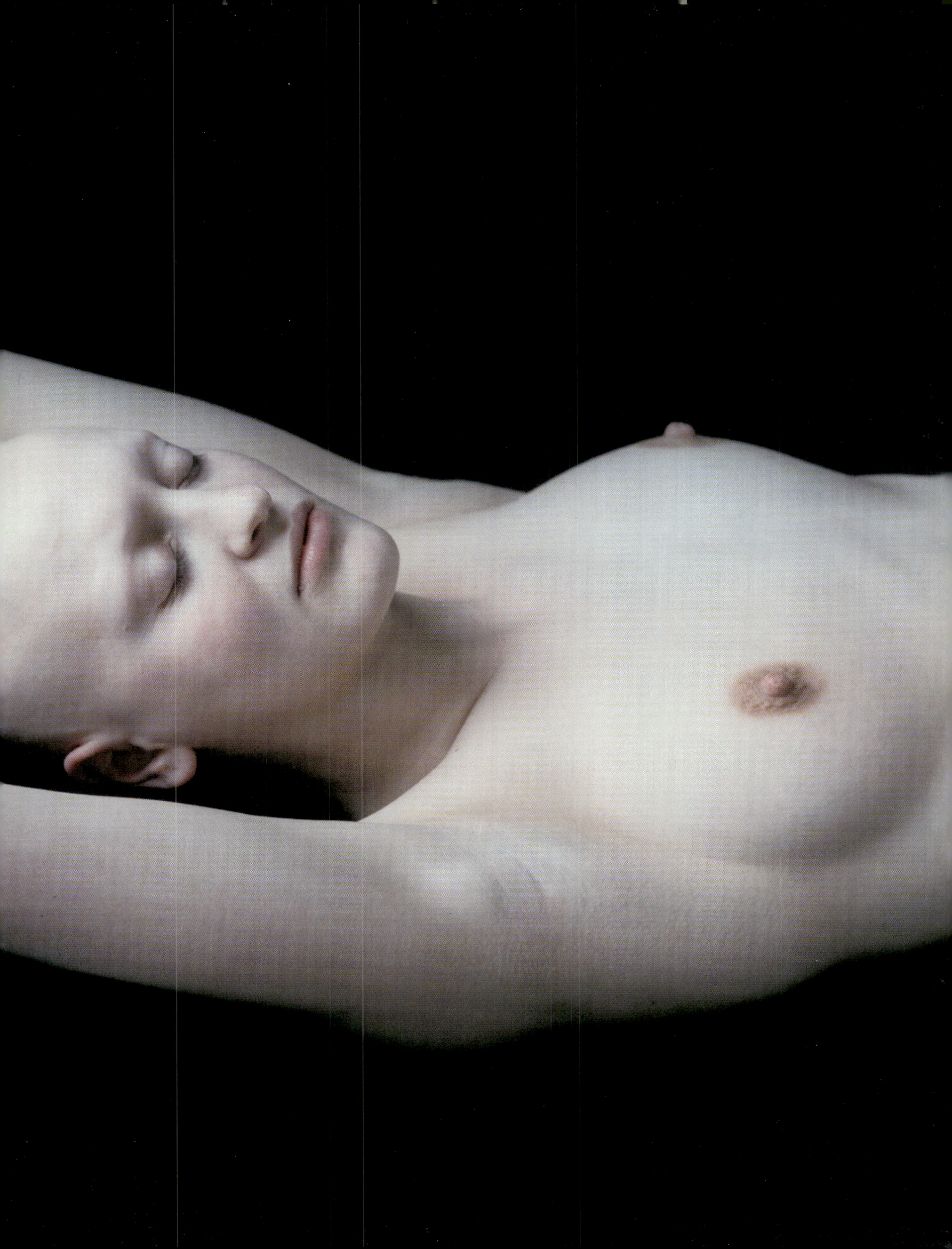

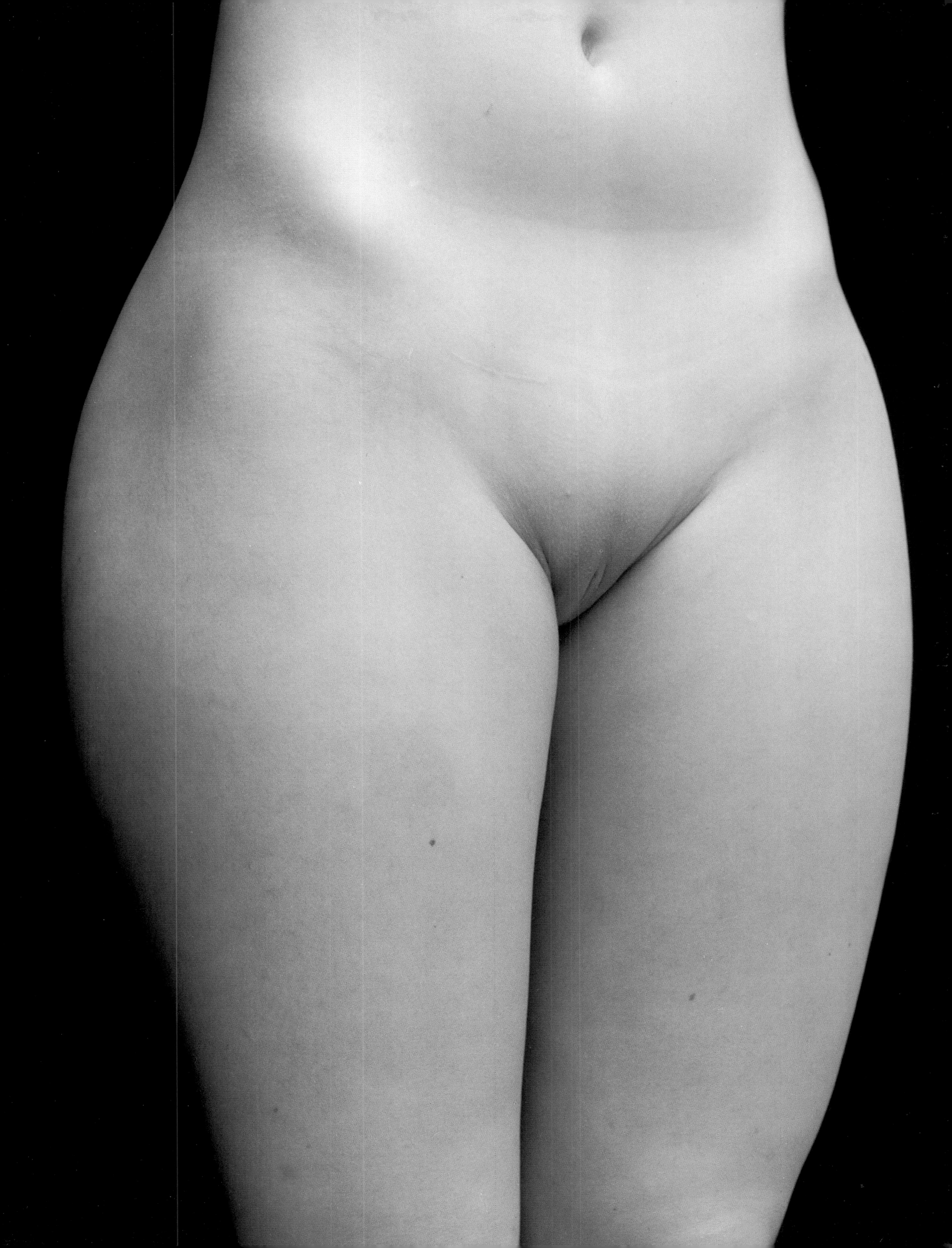

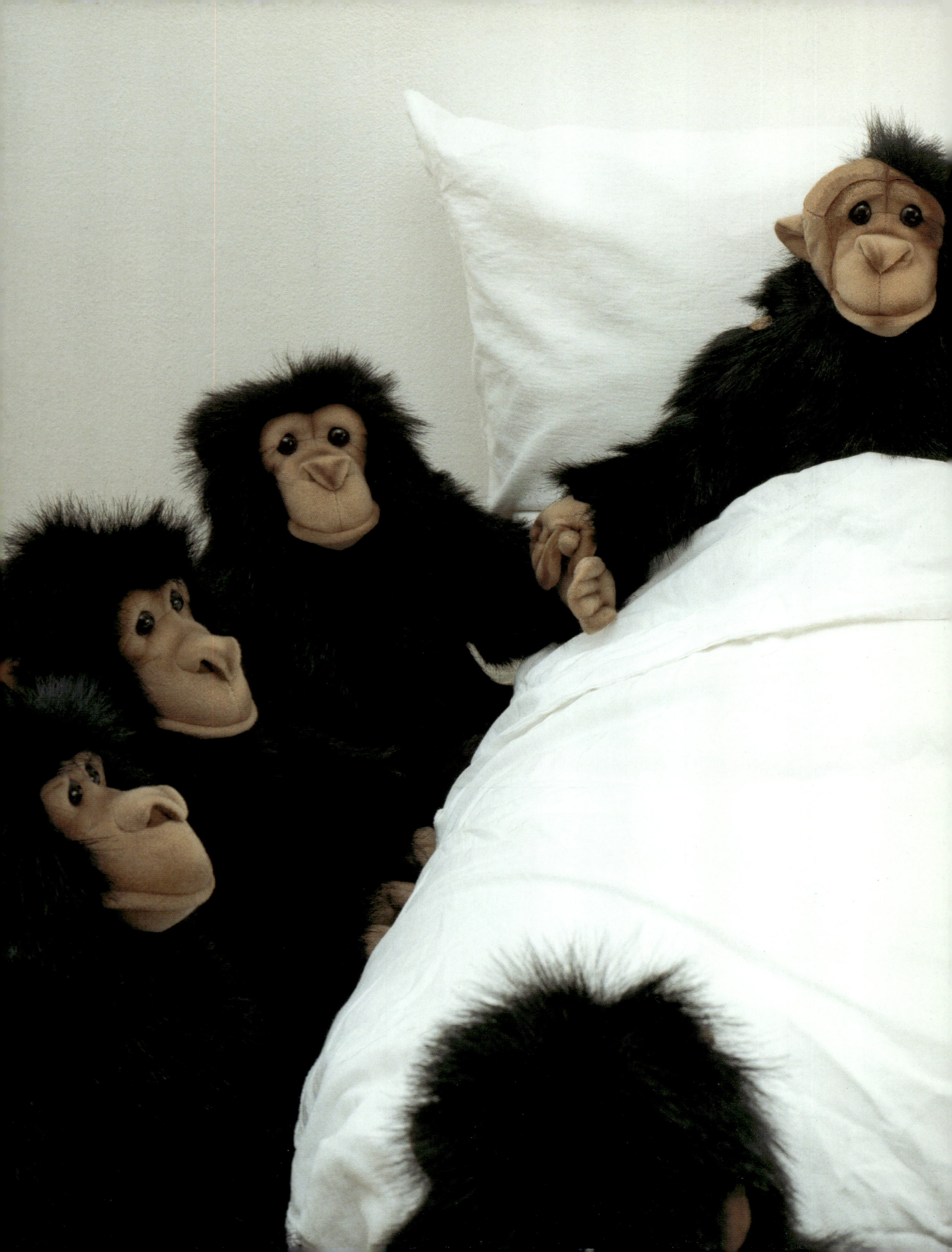

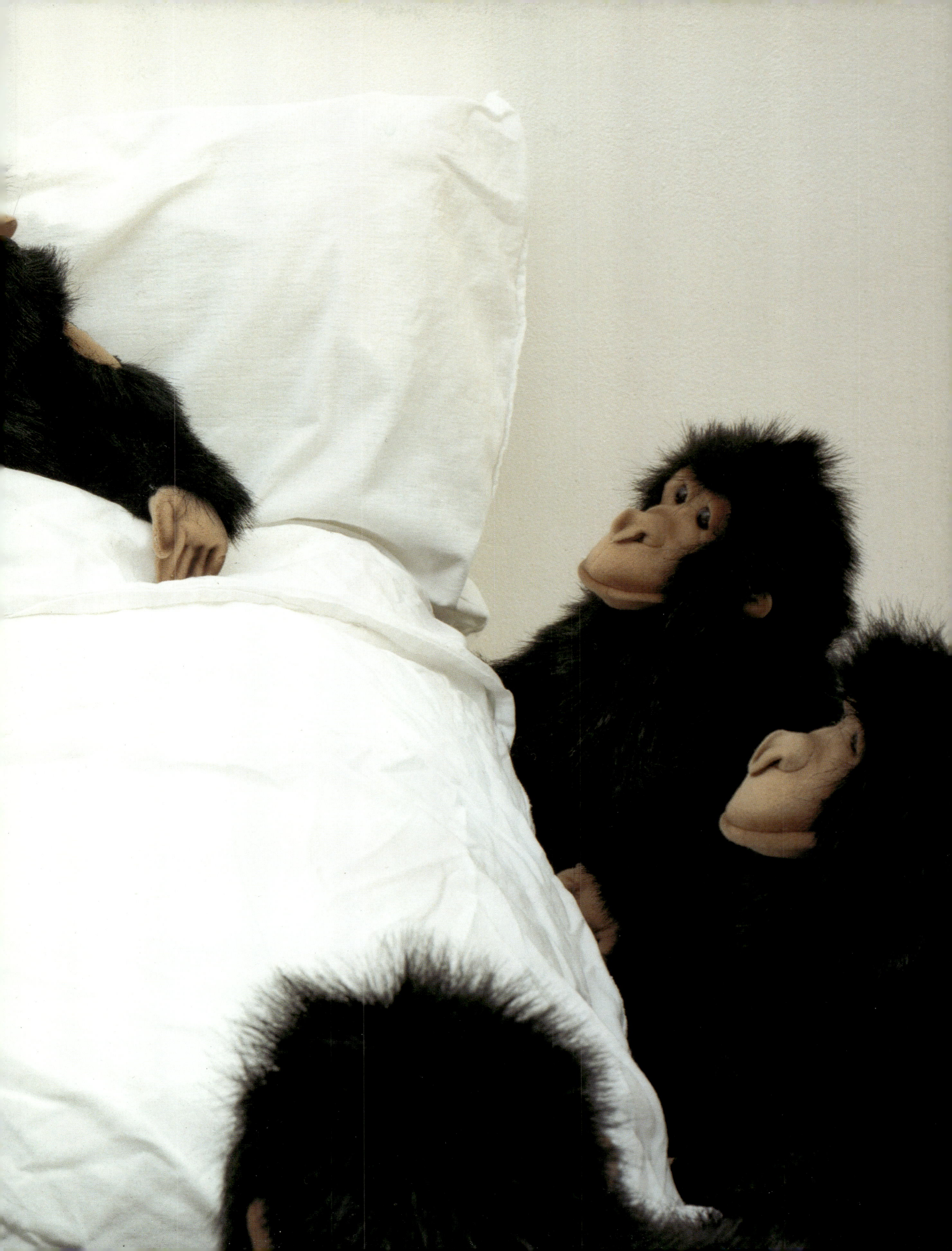

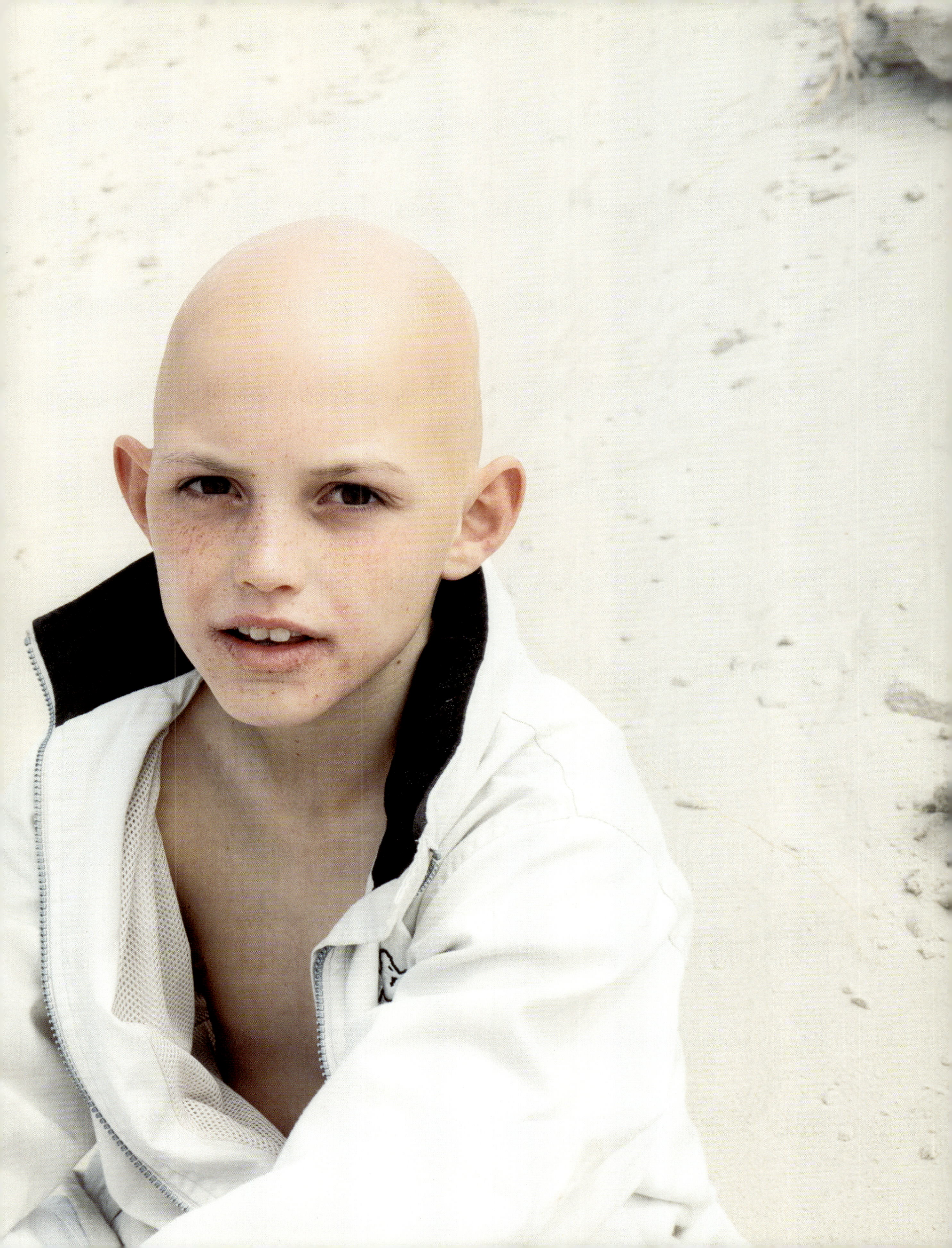

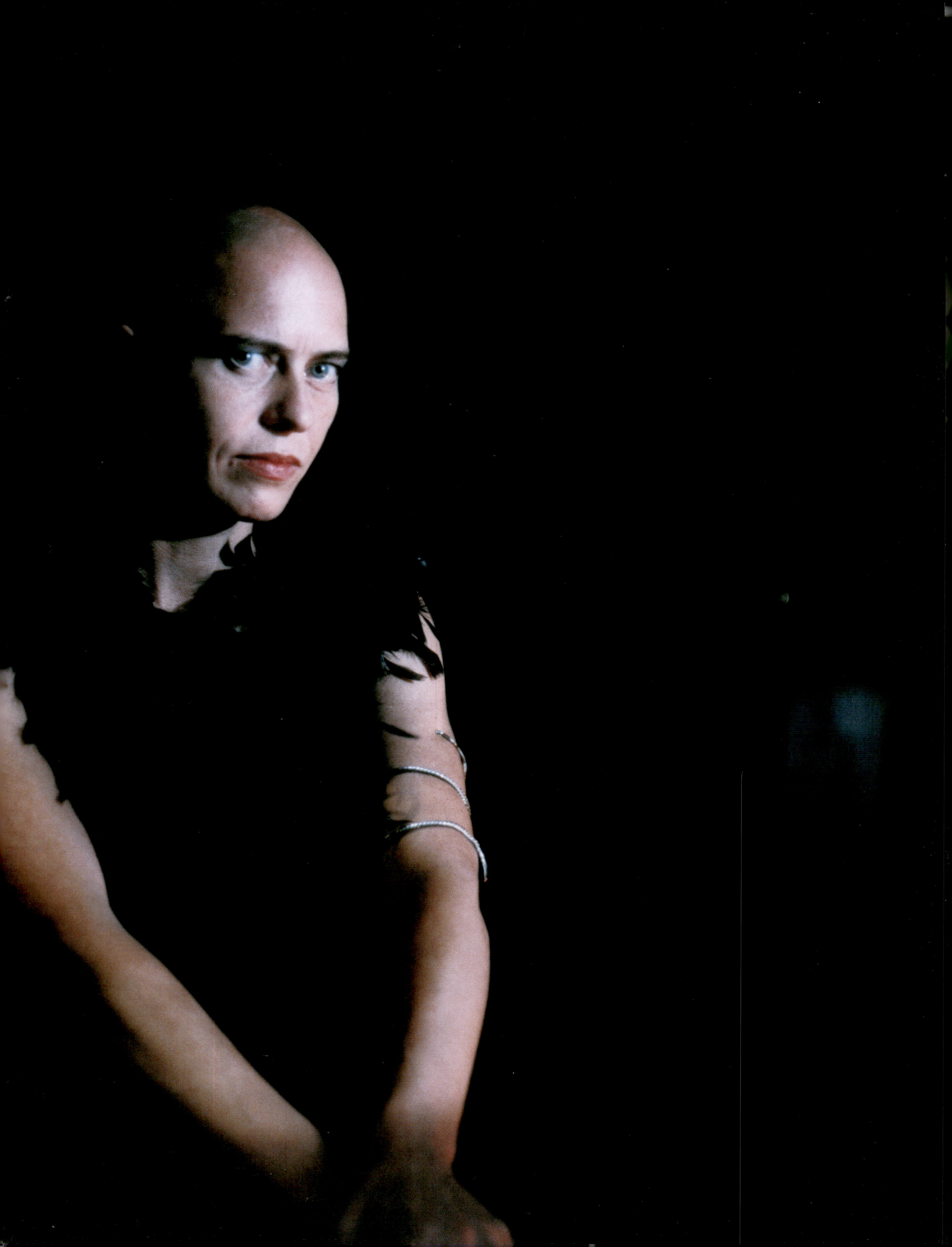

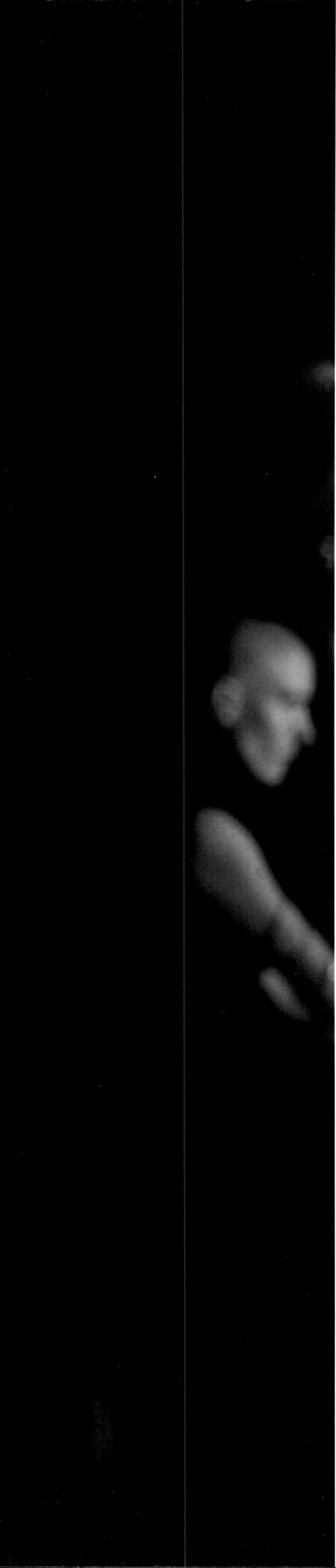

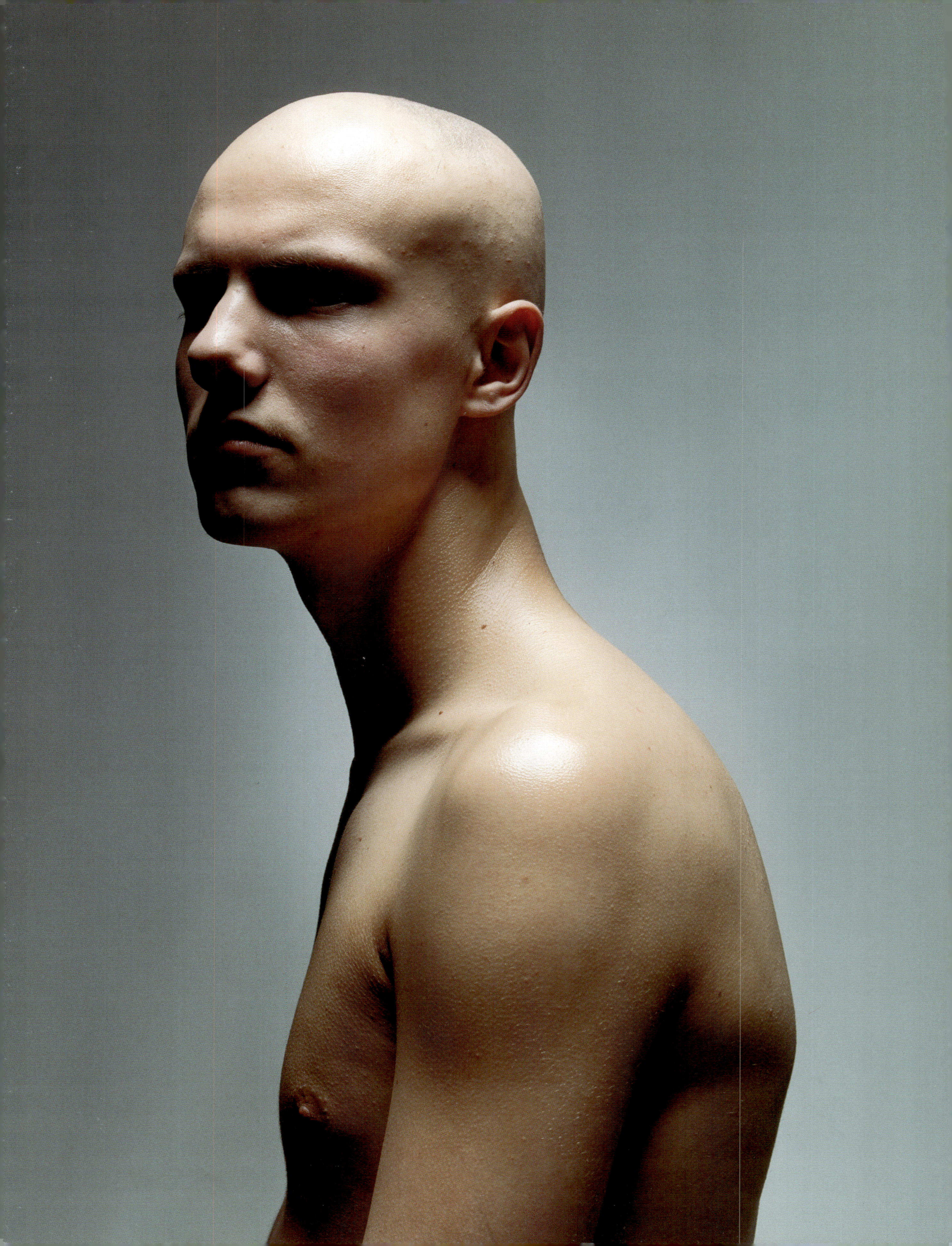

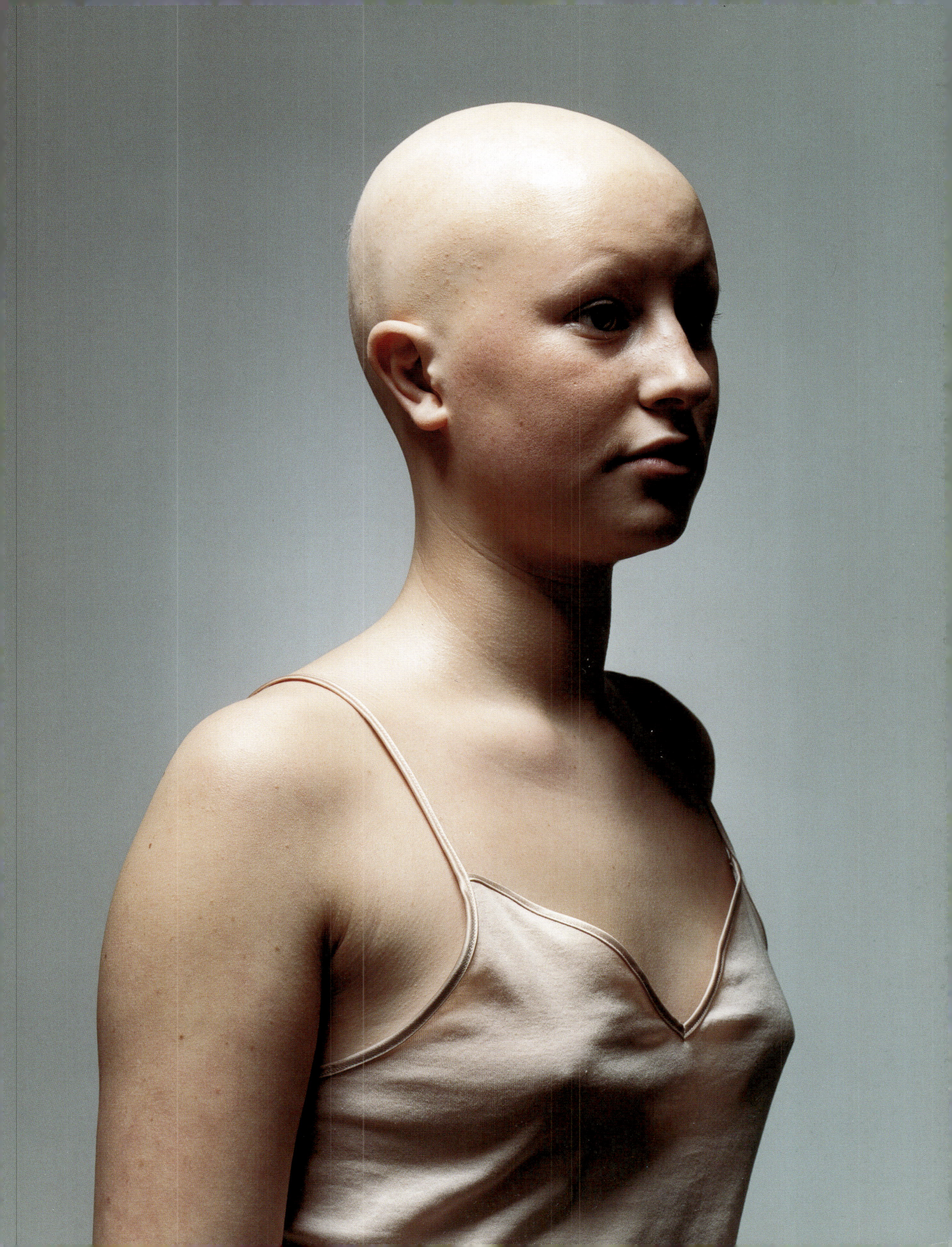

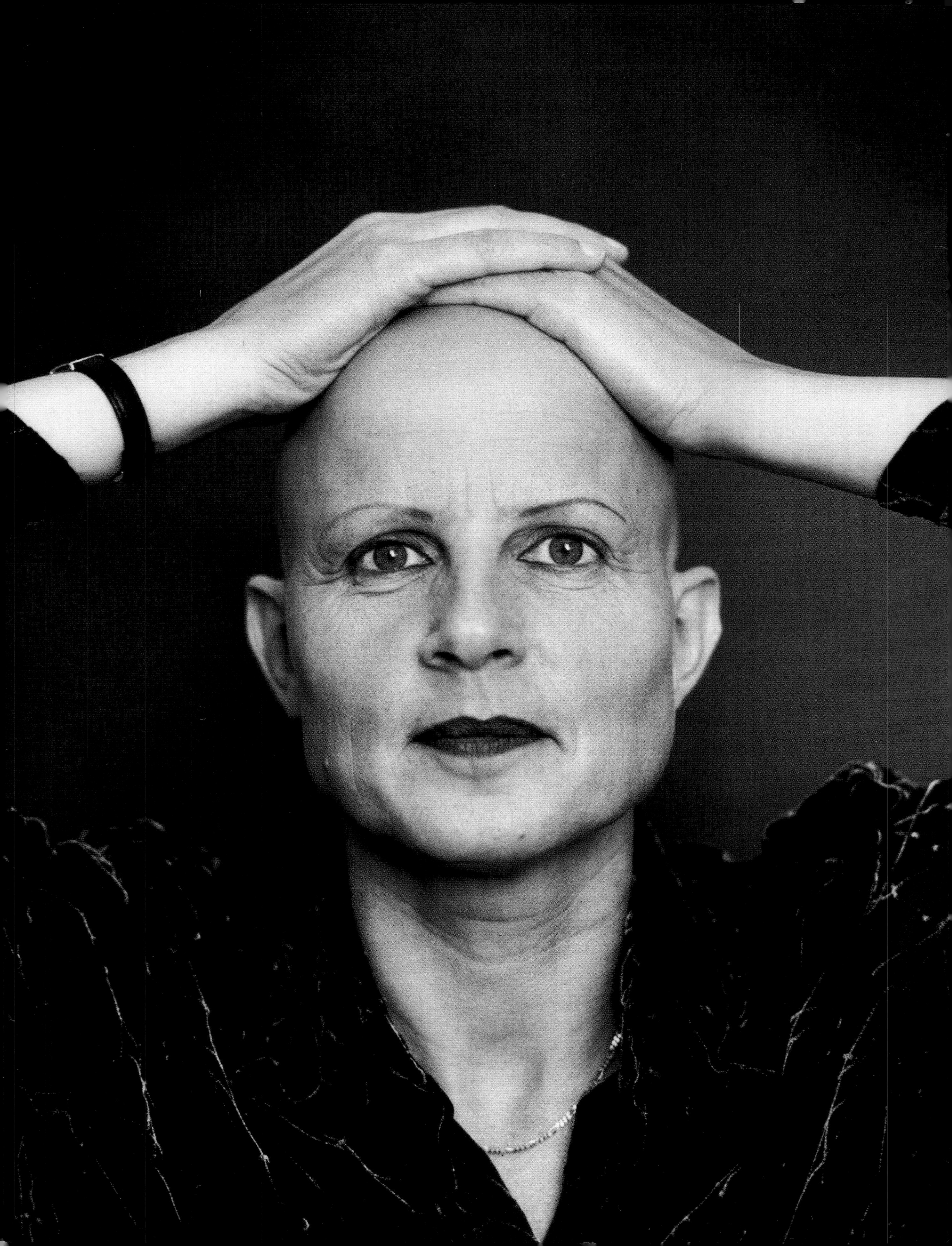

What is alopecia areata?

Professor Jan D. Bos, MD

Alopecia areata literally means patchy (= areata) baldness (= alopecia). The condition can be described as a benign illness of the roots of the hair which results in localised hair loss - generally on the head, but this can also occur on other places on the body. The spots where alopecia occurs are as a rule round or oval. All, or almost all of the hair falls out from these spots, while the surrounding skin shows normal hair growth. As a consequence, one or more bald spots appear in the hair on the head, eyebrows, eyelashes, in the beard, arm-pits or pubic region. In some cases body hair may disappear entirely, and sometimes the nails can also be affected.
It is estimated that 2% of the population will experience alopecia areata for a period at some time in their life. Men and women are equally affected. The first bald spots can appear at any age, even at very early ages, but generally occur before the age of 40.

Alopecia areata is caused by a localised inflammation around the roots of the hair. This inflammation impedes normal hair growth, resulting in the growth of malformed hair which breaks off easily, or no hair growth at all. The roots of the hair are not destroyed by the inflammation. This means that as soon as the inflammation disappears - sometimes after several years - hair growth will resume.
The precise cause of alopecia areata is not known. It is assumed that it is a result of an auto-immune reaction: that is to say, that the body's own immune system identifies parts of the body as outside agents and begins to attack them. Why the immune system malfunctions in this way in some people is unclear. This theory is strengthened by the fact that it appears patients with alopecia areata show an increased frequency of suffering other auto-immune conditions, such as some thyroid diseases, vitiligo and allergic conditions such as eczema and asthma. Psychological factors can also influence the illness. Alopecia areata often appears after a period of increased stress or a profound emotional event. Alopecia areata can also manifest itself after aninfection or after the use of certain medicines. To what extent alopecia areata is hereditary is not known. It is recognised that for about 10% of the patients, the condition has already been identified among other members of their family. Thus there is apparently a certain predisposition to the disease.

The course of alopecia areata is extremely capricious, and differs in each case. It is difficult to predict if and when the hair will return, and whether this recovery will be lasting. Generally - that is to say, in about 80% of the cases - hair growth resumes within a period of several months to a year. In some cases however there will be no total recovery, or hair growth will resume in the original patches, but new bald patches will appear elsewhere. It can also happen that the baldness will spread to extend over the whole head or the entire body. However, the baldness is not by definition irreversible. In principle, it remains possible that hair will return.

The baldness can be a psychological burden for people who have to live with it. In some cases it can lead to serious psycho-social problems which can cause people to become socially isolated.

Alopecia areata is not infectious, and persons who suffer from it can be entirely healthy otherwise.

With thanks to the Nationaal Huidfonds (National Skin Fund)

Pho t og rap her s

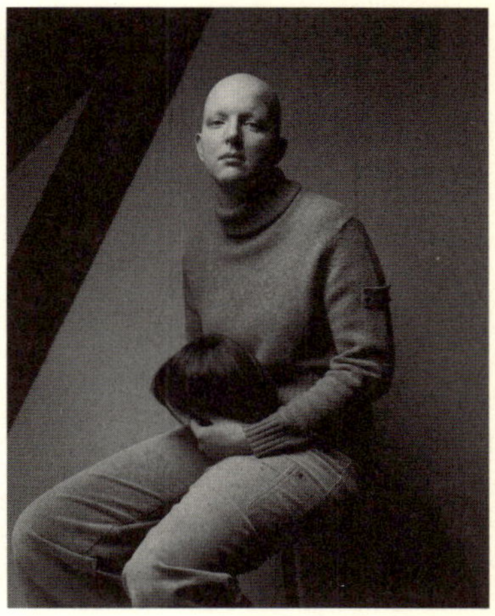

Adrienne M. Norman
Born in Vancouver, 1964
Lives in Amsterdam

Adrienne M. Norman has been living in Amsterdam since 1990 and works primarily as a portrait photographer. In addition to performing assignments from periodicals and organisations, she also photographs for various projects that are connected with particular human themes. In 2000 she published the book Fathers and Daughters on father-daughter relations, and in 2002 she was involved in the publication Heftig Vel by the author Tanny Dobbelaar, for which she did portraits of people who suffer from various skin diseases. The tension between the inward and outward is important in her photographs. For Undercover/ Onthecover she photographed a young woman who never goes out of the house without a wig. Although she dared to be photographed bald, she held on to her wig carefully during the photo session, as a sign of their bond.

Model: Ingmar, age 25
Photo: 60 x 75 cm

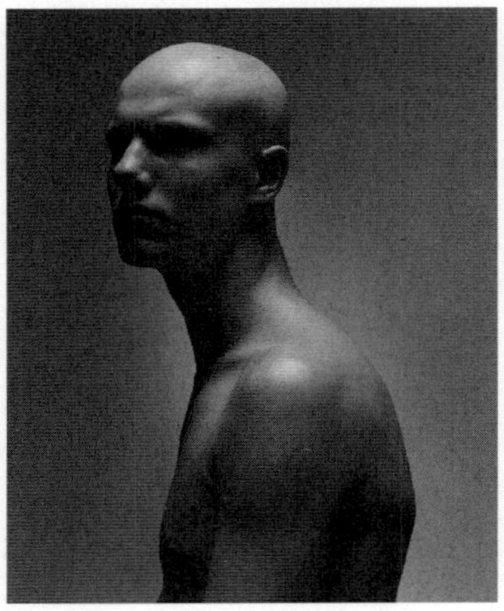

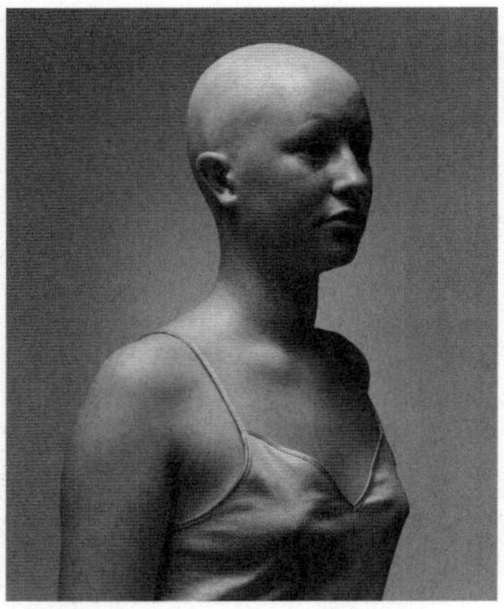

Jouk Oosterhof
Born in Delft, 1973
Lives in Amsterdam

Among Jouk Oosterhof's editorial clients are AD magazine, Elle and Dazed & Confused. In addition to work for periodicals, she is active as an advertising photographer for Nike, Rabobank and Dutch Railways, among others. She has also done poster photographs for the Vagina Monologues, the Over het IJ festival and other theatrical productions. The serenity with wich she portrays her subjects, sometimes with humour, sometimes in a painterly manner, is characteristic of her work. For this project she photographed a boy and a girl in all their baldness and candour. According to Oosterhof, it is important that the personal aura of the subject defines the photograph, and not the illness.

Models: Laura, age 14
and Matthijs, age 16
Photo's: 80 x 100 cm
Agency: edsonwilliams, Amsterdam

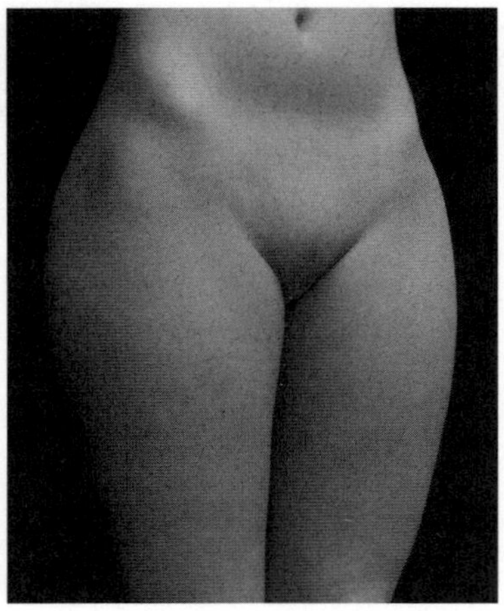

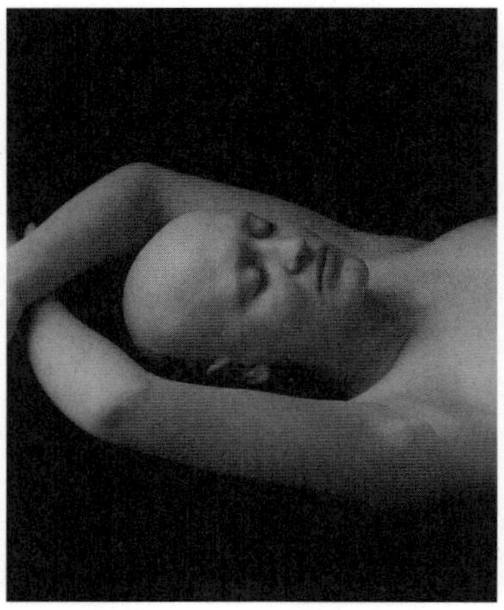

Carla van de Puttelaar
Born in Zaandam, 1967
Lives in Amsterdam

The skin is one of the main themes in the work of Carla van de Puttelaar. She photographs parts of the female body, usually nude. The skin as an area of visual attention is a symbol for feminine aspects such as beauty, sensuality and vulnerability. Except for physical characteristics, Van de Puttelaar leaves individual characteristics out of consideration. Often it is only a scar, the pressure marks from panties or a bruise that contradicts the anonymity of the body. Furthermore, her models have a preternatural white tint because of her use of clear and bright light against a dark background, picking out and emphasising the surface of the skin. The subject she photographed for Undercover/Onthecover appears to fit naturally into Van de Puttelaar's regular work. The nude, hairless body has values that make it both erotically desirable and aesthetically disorienting.

Model: Liselotte, age 21
Photo's: 63 x 77 cm and 77 x 63 cm
Courtesy: Van Zoetendaal, Amsterdam

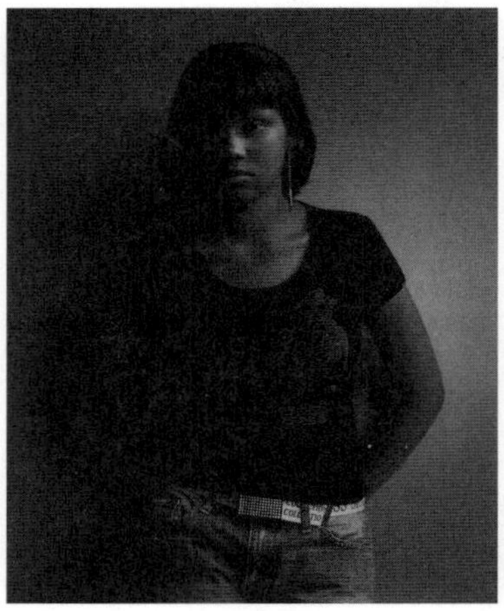

Desiree Dolron
Born in Haarlem, 1963
Lives in Amsterdam

Desiree Dolron combines two different photographic genres. She photographs in the tradition of documentary photography during trips to distant countries, but she also makes staged photographs which she subsequently manipulates digitally. In her portraits she tries to convey the individual's most extreme or striking aspects. In this case she has photographed a young girl who leans casually against a wall while wearing her wig. Without the knowledge that she is hiding her baldness with the wig, it would not be clear that there is anything amiss with her, or that, for instance, she has alopecia areata. This makes the image simultaneously shocking and accusatory: as viewers we are aware that we know something that we really should not know. With this, Dolron draws attention to the tension between objective looking and subjective interpretation.

Model: Nanda, age 13
Photo: 52 x 65 cm
Courtesy: Michael Hoppen, London

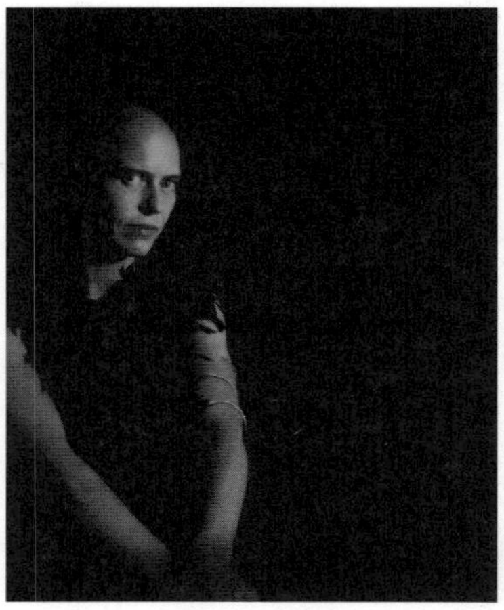

Ine Lamers
Born in Wychen, 1954
Lives in Rotterdam

Ine Lamers works with various media, including photography, video and film, which she shows in a three-dimensional context. The ultimate form of presentation is just as important as the artwork itself. One of the main themes in Lamers's work is the human condition and the relation between people and their surroundings. A human being is a subject and object at the same time, and both looks and is looked at. In Undercover/Onthecover the aspect which particularly fascinated her was that of being looked at, and the projections that people place on others with a aberrant or unusual appearance. With the aid of the photograph of her model she wants to 'provoke a process of consciousness-raising in the viewer, so that the viewer consciously "undergoes" the process of looking and reflects on his or her own projections during that looking. In other words: the viewer should become aware of his or her own glasses or filter.'

Model: Margriet, age 36
Photo: 110 x 110 cm

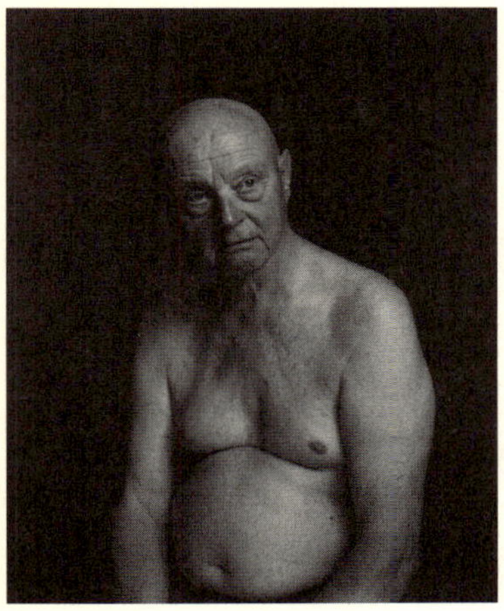

Koos Breukel

Born in The Hague, 1962
Lives in Amsterdam

'Existential' is a term often used for the portraits by Koos Breukel. His subjects, photographed at an unguarded moment, appear lost in thought and turned in upon themselves. Breukel works with great sensitivity for his subject, in black and white with a traditional view camera which renders them in razor-sharp detail against a dark background. As well as the individuality of the person, traces that the life they have lived have left upon them are to be found in the picture. That has also occurred with the person he photographed for Undercover/Onthecover. Looking closely, it can be seen in the extremely detailed image that the older man is not only entirely bald, but that he has no eyelashes or eyebrows, nor any other body hair. However confrontational it is, the ageing body of his model and his hairlessness emphasise his inseparable connection with life.

Model: Geert, age 77
Photo: 100 x 120 cm
Courtesy: Van Zoetendaal, Amsterdam

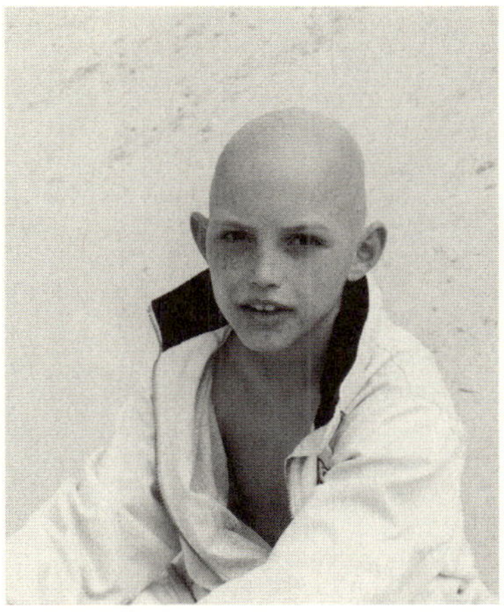

Noor Damen

Born in Deventer, 1949
Lives in Uitdam

Noor Damen has occupied herself with photography since 1970; before that she worked as a designer for theatre costumes, and designed clothing for various Dutch dance groups. The essence of being human is central in her photographs. Through the outward form she tries to say something about the content, or to lay bare the underlying layers which are not visible at first glance. She also did this in photographing young Steven, whose illness is clearly visible. With this photograph Damen emphasises the tension which can arise between an individual's outward appearance and how the person himself feels. By making alopecia areata visible and discussible, she hopes to bring this disease out of its isolation.

Model: Steven, age 12
Photo: 80 x 100 cm
Courtesy: Van Kranendonk, The Hague

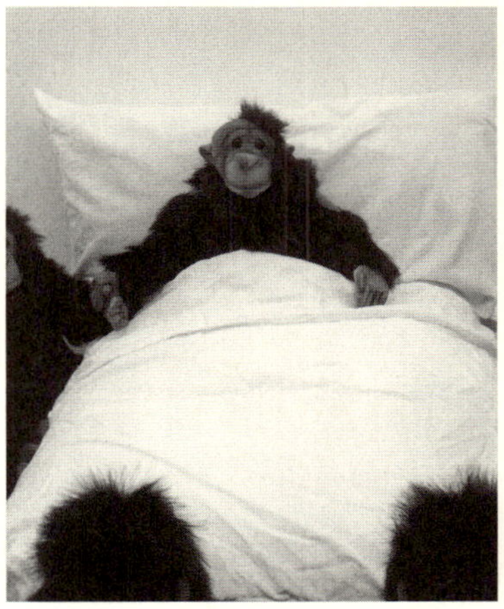

Bert Sissingh

Born in The Hague, 1956
Lives in Rotterdam

Irony and humour are two important aspects in the work of Bert Sissingh. He is primarily known for family portraits in which he and his parents figure, and apparently everyday occurrences are re-enacted. In the role of the eternal child, he depicts his relation to his parents, in which traditional role patterns, old norms and values are central. In visualising alopecia areata, he deliberately opted not to use a model. With the assistance of toy monkeys Sissingh represents the situation of the patient and his or her acquaintances in a remarkable manner: the patient who does not feel ill sees his or her situation become all the more unbearable through the patronising concern of others. Sissingh's photograph serves as a statement to the public at large and at the same time to give heart to patients.

In co-operation with Sjoukje Boersma
Photo: 80 x 100 cm

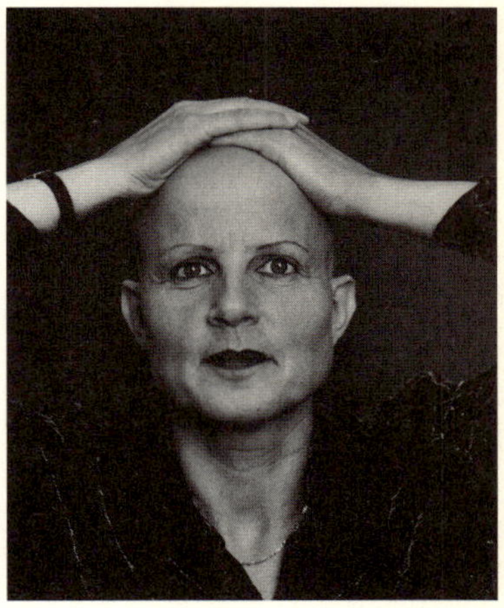

Vincent Mentzel

Born in Hoogkarspel, 1945
Lives in Rotterdam

Since the 1970s Vincent Mentzel has worked for the NRC Handelsblad. Beginning as a photo reporter, today he is one of the best-known photojournalists in the Netherlands. His easy manner with people assures that he can get them to pose for him without difficulty. He has done portraits of many politicians, national and international celebrities, and members of the Royal House. Later he got the opportunity to travel and prepared many photo essays for M Magazine and other publications. Accustomed to making photographs which are above all informative, he found it an unusual experience to co-operate on Undercover/Onthecover. With a feeling for the vulnerability of the model, he photographed her while she both exposes herself and partially covers herself with her hands.

Model: Ida, age 48
Photo: 100 x 100 cm

Photography
Noor Damen
Ine Lamers
Desiree Dolron
Koos Breukel
Carla van de Puttelaar
Jouk Oosterhof
Vincent Mentzel
Adrienne M. Norman
Bert Sissingh
(with Sjoukje Boersma)

Coverphoto
Wim van Egmond

Initiator and Concept
Monique Benthin
SAM Stichting Art Medicine

Text
Marijn van der Jagt
artjournalist
Claudia Küssel
Nederlands fotomuseum
Prof. Dr Jan D. Bos
National Skin Fund

Editor
Frits Gierstberg
Nederlands fotomuseum

Translation
Donald Mader

Graphic Design
-SYB- Utrecht

Printing and Lithography
Die Keure, Brugge, Belgium

Exposition
The accompanying exhibition takes place from 5 March till 17 April 2005, Nederlands fotomuseum, Rotterdam (see www.nederlandsfotomuseum.nl).

Financial support
Mondriaanstichting
VSB fonds
Rotterdamse Kunststichting
Centrum Beeldende Kunst
SBAW
Nederlands fotomuseum

Publisher
Artimo - Gijs Stork
Elandsgracht 8
1016 TV Amsterdam
t +31 20 625 3344
info@artimo.net

Distribution
D.A.P.
155 Sixth Avenue, 2nd floor
NY 10013 New York
t +1 212 627 1999
dap@dapinc.com

Idea Books
Nieuwe Herengracht 11
1011 RK Amsterdam
t +31 20 622 6154
idea@ideabooks.nl

Art Data
12 Bell Industrial Estate,
50 Cunnington Street
W4 5HB London
t +44 20 8747 1061
info@artdata.co.uk

ISBN
90-8546-028-X